Simply Keto Diet For Weight Loss Practical Guide

How To Lose 20 Healthy Pounds in 30 Days with 30 Delicious Proven Ketogenic

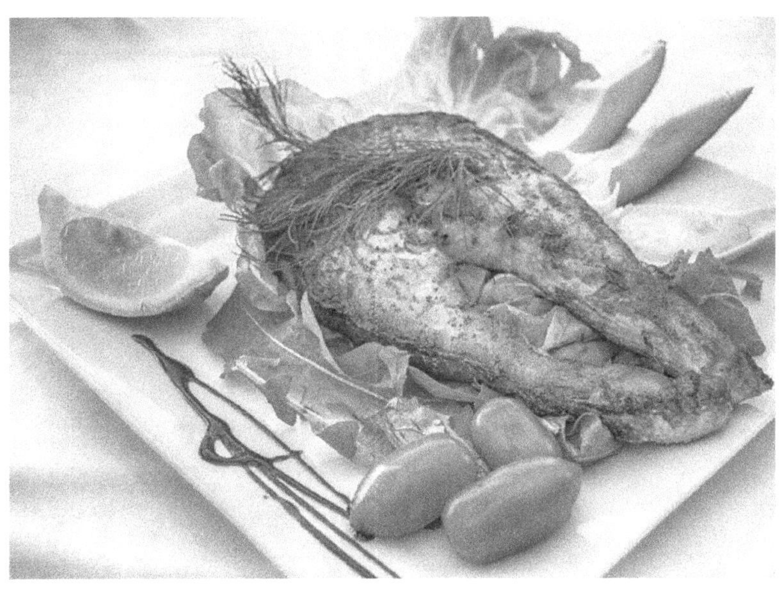

Paul Ketony

ISBN: 9781797454634

Legal & Disclaimer

The information contained in this book and its contents is not designed to replace or take the place of any form of medical or professional advice; and is not meant to replace the need for independent medical, financial, legal or other professional advice or services, as may be required. The content and information in this book has been provided for educational and entertainment purposes only.

The content and information contained in this book has been compiled from sources deemed reliable, and it is accurate to the best of the Author's knowledge, information and belief. However, the Author cannot guarantee its accuracy and validity and cannot be held liable for any errors and/or omissions. Further, changes are periodically made to this book as and when needed. Where appropriate and/or necessary, you must consult a professional (including but not limited to your doctor, attorney, financial advisor or such other professional advisor) before using any of the suggested remedies, techniques, or information in this book.

Upon using the contents and information contained in this book, you agree to hold harmless the Author from and against any damages, costs, and expenses, including any legal fees potentially resulting from the application of any of the information provided by this book. This disclaimer applies to any loss, damages or injury caused by the use and application, whether directly or indirectly, of any advice or information presented, whether for breach of contract, tort, negligence, personal injury, criminal intent, or under any other cause of action.

You agree to accept all risks of using the information presented inside this book.

You agree that by continuing to read this book, where appropriate and/or necessary, you shall consult a professional (including but not limited to your doctor, attorney, or financial advisor or such other advisor as needed) before using any of the suggested remedies, techniques, or information in this book.

CONTENTS

INTRODUCTION

Obesity has become a global epidemic, due to changes in the diet that the population has suffered, mainly because of the lack of time to which it is subjected, as a result of a modern and hectic life.

Chronic diseases that were previously thought to be typical of adults are now are being alarmingly diagnosed in the smallest.

The ketogenic diet is a diet that has been scientifically proven, based on actual results. It began to be implemented in 1920, specifically in the hospital Johns Hopkins, in patients in the area of neurosurgery and neurology, giving excellent results.

After observing the results of the ketogenic diet obtained in this first stage, it was adopted to improve the health conditions of various chronic diseases and as an effective method to lose weight.

Currently, it is a diet widely used by the world population that struggles with the problems of overweight and diseases arising from it. Its success is due to the fact that it is healthy, easy to follow and does not impose limits.

This book has been created especially for people who want to improve their physical and mental conditions, as well as diminish effects and avoid diseases caused by obesity or overweight.

It contains 30 delicious recipes, easy and quick to prepare the ketogenic diet, which are perfectly combinable with the recommended foods.

Empower yourself with knowledge and break the myth about the ketogenic diet. Learn to eat healthily, prepare your dishes easily, cheaply, without starvation or expose yourself to great sacrifices.

Dieting should not be synonymous with limitations; it is about applying the right knowledge in food preparation.

Invest in health and find out how to make your metabolism work for you!

CHAPTER I

WHAT IS THE KETO DIET?

It is a useful technique of combining macronutrients contained in food, which is used in order to modify the metabolic behavior of the body and achieve the use of fats in reserve as energy.

It is about re-educating the organism through the modification of eating habits aimed at promoting weight loss and improving people's quality of life.

The main characteristic of this diet is that it is low in carbohydrates, with high levels of "good" fats with a significant percentage of protein and fiber.

This combination of macronutrients changes the function of metabolism, producing an induced state of ketosis, which makes use of fats in reserves found in the body, due to the lack of carbohydrate intake.

It occurs with the ketogenic diet, a similar process in the body when fasting. The human body is programmed to resolve by itself the lack of energy supply contained in carbohydrates.

When the supply of carbohydrates is not sufficient, the metabolism turns to fat reserves to convert them into an energy source.

Types

There are several types of ketogenic diets:

Standard: 75% fat, 20% protein and 5% carbohydrates of good quality and with lots of fiber.

Directed: adopted by athletes and allows adding carbohydrates in training periods.

High in protein: 60% fat, 35% protein and 5% carbohydrates of good quality and high fiber. This diet is used in special conditions such as pregnancy, postpartum, people who want to develop muscles and those who for some reason require increased protein intake.

Cyclic: it is combined; 5 days ketogenic and 2 days with high consumption in carbohydrates. Bodybuilders use it.

In each particular case, the amount of food must be modified.

In this EBook, we will deal with the **standard ketogenic diet** because it is the most used diet in the population.

This diet has the particularity that adapts to the needs and conditions of each person. The results obtained are according to the modifications you make in the quantity of food, within the ketogenic diet.

In Western culture, more than 250 grams of carbohydrates are consumed in the daily diet, generally refined, including sugars.

How it works

A person whose daily requirement is 2000 calories, his carbohydrate intake should be between 50 and 100 grams distributed in the meals of the day.

It is recommended that you approach the lower limit for best results, which is 50 grams or less.

The body by receiving a lower amount of carbohydrates activates the production of ketones and causes a decrease in glucose in the blood, as it is taking the body reserves to transform them into energy.

Ketones go into the bloodstream and produce a series of symptoms typical of ketosis.
This natural process results in a considerable decrease of ketones in the blood, which translates into weight loss and other health benefits.

How do you know if you're in ketosis?

The process of adaptation of the ketogenic diet takes about 2 weeks, in this period occur mild changes and symptoms that disappear on their own, and with which the body gives you clues that your body has entered ketosis.

There are several ways to know if you are in ketosis:

Ketone breath:

Fruity or metallic odor on the third day of the start of the diet.

Dry mouth and increased thirst:

This phenomenon occurs with the elimination of sodium, potassium, and water through urine. (Drink liquids).

Ketone in urine

It can be proven by laboratory tests or the use of commercially available urine ketone measuring strips.

Ketones in blood:

It is reliable, in laboratory examination.

It is essential to evaluate the process very carefully, weight loss should be stabilized around the 10th and 12th week, and there may be variations in each particular case.

Benefits

You learn to eat healthily
Slimming.
Increased self-esteem.
Increased energy.
Mental Agility.
Longevity.
Decrease in the risk of disease.
Physical performance.
Safety.
Sensation of general well-being.

It has been scientifically proven that the ketogenic diet decreases and slows down the effects of diseases such as diabetes, cancer, epilepsy, Alzheimer's disease, Parkinson's disease, ovarian cysts, acne, gastritis, brain damage, among others, and prevents other diseases resulting from obesity.

CHAPTER II

REASONS FOR THE REBOUND EFFECT?

Psychological

The main cause for the rebound effect in 98% of cases is in mind. When starting a diet plan, it is essential to have a firm determination to achieve the goals you have set.

You must assume with all responsibility and discipline the changes and challenges you face when starting your diet. There are many mental factors involved in the process of weight loss, and we will discuss them later.

In many cases, the same person blocks himself as a result of low self-esteem. It is necessary to sweep these obstacles from your mind and be prepared for success.

On the other hand, some specialists believe that the lack of follow-up is one of the causes of the rebound effect; however, it is unlikely that there is a lifetime follow-up in a diet.

For this reason is that each person should monitor and control their own progress, this can only be achieved with a firm decision to change and follow a pre-established plan to obtain definitive results.

Miracle Diets

Those diets that are promoted in the mainstream media and that promise miracles usually cause the person a state of frustration and depression to see that the results are adverse to what they expected.

Currently, there are several products on the market such as tea, injections, patches, pills, and others, which should be observed with great caution.

Many people confuse their body's responses to the diet or treatment they have adopted with weight loss, ending up affecting their health and in worse conditions than they were before starting the so-called "miraculous" diet.

Limitations

Diets that impose limits and sacrifices on you are doomed to failure. If you feel limited to tasting what you want, sooner or later you end up giving up and abandoning your dream of seeing yourself thin.

It is common to hear obese people say, "I am fat but happy," this is because they are not forbidden to enjoy one of the best pleasures of life as it is to eat.

The ketogenic diet allows the ingestion of the majority of foods, only demands responsibility in the quantities and a lot of discipline.

Habits

The change of habits is essential at the time of initiating the ketogenic diet; most people fail because they neglect the practice of habits beneficial to the diet.

The habits are strengthened day by day, the practice turns them into automatic acts of our daily life as breathing, walking and do not need any effort.

Lifestyle

To experience healthy physical and mental changes, it is essential to change your lifestyle; without it, you can't transform your own reality.

If you change the way you live and start from within, your reality becomes transformed, empowered and allows you to take control of your life.

Compare yourself with others.

Each individual is unique and responds differently to the same treatment, for this reason, it is essential to be attentive to the signals your body sends you and to know yourself.

Thinking that a diet will have the same effects on you as the results it gave your friend is a mistake that many people make and end up frustrated, depressed and recovering even more of the weight loss.

CHAPTER III

FACTORS TO CONSIDER BEFORE STARTING A KETO DIET

Health

You should consult your physician before starting the ketogenic diet plan, to obtain favorable results. It is essential to be in good health to initiate a change in eating habits.

There is an initial stage of adaptation of the organism to the ketogenic diet, which lasts approximately 2 weeks. During this period of adaptation, you will feel changes in the body that should not alarm you; it is only indicating that you have entered a state of ketosis.

Time

Time is an essential factor to take into account, especially for those who work and have little time to take care of their food.

The selection and preparation of food is recommended that you do it yourself since only you are a guarantee that you will choose the best quality.

Exercise routine

Exercise at least 3 times a week to supplement your diet, stay active, oxygenate your brain and improve your mood. If you don't have time to exercise, at least walk 30 minutes daily.

Other

Be honest with yourself, follow your plan and make a firm decision to transform your reality.

CHAPTER IV

ANCESTRAL TECHNIQUES TO KNOW THE TYPE OF FOOD THAT GOES WITH YOUR METABOLISM.

Since ancient times, food has been considered the primary source of energy for life. Secrets of longevity are revealed, which are achieved by applying techniques to find and rescue balance in harmony with nature.
They affirm that diets should be in accordance with each person's type of metabolism for best results.

According to the outstanding philosophers several centuries A of C, there are two types of metabolisms, slow oxidation, and rapid oxidation. The slow oxidation metabolism easily processes and assimilates foods of plant origin, and the fast oxidation metabolism easily digests foods of animal origin, sugars, and carbohydrates.

To find out what type of metabolism a body has, the meat technique (eating a large amount of red or white meat) is tested and the behavior of the body is evaluated. If the person feels mental discomfort or stomach heaviness, it is said to be slow oxidation.

It is essential to know how to identify the type of metabolism that you have to select your diet correctly.

Natural approach

To look for foods in their natural state, to preserve the health and to avoid the evils product of toxic agents contained in industrialized foods.

They recommend consuming food in its natural state, preferably not long after it has been harvested, avoiding the use of fertilizers and chemicals to preserve it. Avoid processed, canned or canned foods.

The meat should be from animals that have not suffered mistreatment, and their feeding has been of high quality.

The above conditions guarantee the energy that releases each food, as well as the influence that each flavor and color has on each of the organs of the human body, necessary to define the health and longevity of each individual.

CHAPTER V

GUIDE TO DEVELOP THE PLAN THAT SUITS THE NEEDS OF YOUR BODY

Action plan

From the very moment you decide to start your ketogenic diet, you must draw up your action plan. Establish in a systematic way and by hierarchy each one of the tasks or small objectives that you must fulfill to achieve your goal of losing weight.

Make a list of all the tasks you perform throughout the 24 hours of the day. Don't forget to include your hours of sleep (8 hours), hours to feed yourself, to buy food and prepare it, to work, to enjoy with your family, to exercise, to relax and to have fun. It includes all the day tasks and assigns a prudential time for the fulfillment of each one.

Goal

Honesty in setting goals is important. You must set goals that you can achieve. It is advisable to start with small goals and as you move forward with your goals, set more demanding goals to avoid frustration and depression.

Objectives

Each of the small steps that must be done systematically and that forge the way to reach your goal of losing weight.

Create, reinforce and change habits

The daily practices of the different actions that benefit the fulfillment of the nutritional plan that you have adopted, are building a solid path, that with the passing of time is part of your daily life and you will hardly change it.

Among the habits that you must create or reinforce are:

- Prepare your food.
- Chew food very well.

- Avoid consuming food with extreme temperatures.
- Choose natural foods.
- Frequent people with the same concerns and that make you feel motivated.
- Listen to good music.
- Reward yourself with the clothes you always wanted to wear.
- Celebrate your triumphs.
- Read a good book.

Eliminate habits that hinder the achievement of your goals:

- Sweets.
- Drugs.
- Smoking.
- Alcoholic beverages.
- To interrupt the nocturnal sleep.
- Procrastination.
- Consumption of sugary drinks.
- Reward yourself with food.
- Learn to say no when others offer you food or drinks that go against your diet.
- Avoid feeling overwhelmed or stressed.

Evaluate tasks at the end of the day to make sure they are done. The process should be evaluated every week, eliminating what has not worked, reinforcing and improving those tasks that have worked.

CHAPTER VI

HOW TO ACHIEVE RESULTS THAT LAST OVER TIME?

Perseverance

Being persistent in your goals, not abandoning your dreams, giving your best to achieve them and finally feel a full satisfaction and a sense of inner well-being, is the closest thing to happiness.

Feeling that you are capable and that you meet the goals you set will make you feel, and your self-esteem remains at its highest level.

Discipline

No one successful person on earth is undisciplined.

The person who develops the capacity for self-control can easily overcome the obstacles that arise along the way towards the fulfillment of their objectives. A disciplined person is a virtuous person.

Managing time

Efficiently manage time, distribute 24 hours a day, assigning each task the estimated time for completion, ensures success in meeting your goals.

Manage your life so that you can assign the necessary time to each thing, according to the degree of importance in your life and avoid feeling overwhelmed.

Organization

The organization allows increasing efficiency levels; tasks become lighter, time and money is saved. The organization decreases errors by a large percentage.

CHAPTER VII

CORRECT FOOD SELECTION AND COMBINATION

Very few foods are banned in the ketogenic diet. It is essential that the person is informed about how metabolism works with this diet and consumes the amounts of food responsibly. Especially those containing carbohydrates.

Daily practice helps you to become familiar with the quantities and substitute foods with the same nutritional value in order to make the food plan more flexible, not to fall into boredom and enjoy the delights of good eating.

The selection of quality foods, the knowledge of the macronutrients contained in each of them and the nutritional needs of each individual are the basis for obtaining the desired results.

The consumption of foods with low carbohydrate content and high fiber content is essential.

1 serving equals 15 grams of carbohydrates.

1 cup of cereal, fruits, legumes, milk or yogurt.
1 slice of bread or a medium tortilla.
1/2 cup oatmeal, 1/3 cup rice.
1/2 cup casserole, 1/2 English muffin, 1/2 cup black beans.
½ cup starchy vegetables, 1/4 of a potato.
2/3 cup plain yogurt.
4 chicken nuggets.
1/2 cup casserole or 1 cup soup.

These foods are equivalent to 1 serving of CARBS

1 Apple, 1 ½ Kiwi, watermelon, ¾ cup Pineapple, blackberries, cherries, 1 Mango, mandarin, orange, guava. 1 Fig, ½ Pear, Peach, Plum, 1 Banana, 1 cup Strawberries, Blackberries, Papaya, Raspberries, Melon or Grapes.

1 cup natural yogurt, liquid skim milk or 4 tablespoons powder.

½ cup chickpeas, beans, lentils, or peas (cooked) or chickpeas.

Medium baked corn tortilla, ¼ cup white rice, and ½ cup boiled potato, natural oatmeal or corn.
1/3 cup amaranth or sweet potato.
1 slice of whole wheat bread.

Coconut or almond bread, 3 tablespoons natural granola or 8 tablespoons wheat bran.

Risks you are exposed to in the ketogenic diet, if there is no control in the measures of macronutrients, according to the needs of your body:

Lipotoxicity; produced by a high consumption of fats. Keep saturated fats below 7%.

Overeating protein; it suspends the state of ketosis and does not affect the diet.

Excessive exercise; produces changes in metabolism and stops the state of ketosis.

❖ It is essential to maintain a balanced proportion of healthy fats, proteins, fibers, and carbohydrates.

Healthy Fats

- Avocado, vegetable oils of canola, avocado, coconut, and olive.
- Eggs.
- Cheeses.
- Butter.
- Walnut seeds.
- Almonds.
- Pumpkin, sunflower, peanut or pistachio seeds.
- Chia, Flaxseed.
- High-fat fish, sardines, tuna, salmon, herring, trout.
- Vinaigrettes based on canola, olive or avocado oils.

Food allowed:

- Protein: lean white, pink and red meats, fish, low-fat cheese, shrimp, turkey, duck, broths, etc.

- Green and starch-free vegetables: nuts, mushrooms, spinach, broccoli, cauliflower, beet, onion, tomatoes, peppers, carrots, turnips, avocado, coconut, seeds, among others.

Foods that must be consumed in a responsible and controlled manner.

- - Pasta, dark chocolate, milk, pizza, wheat flour, bread, biscuits, toast, beans, chickpeas, wholemeal bread, lentils, potatoes, peas, corn, pumpkin, semolina, oats, brown rice, etc.

Avoid consumption of:

- Soft drinks, alcoholic beverages, chocolates, cakes, sweets, fruits with high glucose content, sugary drinks, among others.

- The food can be accompanied by smoothies, flavored water without sugar, coffee, among others.

- Consume daily 3 or 4 fruits of low glucose content and high fiber content.

CHAPTER VIII

30 DELICIOUS KETO RECIPES, EASY AND QUICK FOR PEOPLE WITH LIMITED TIME (PREPARATION 20 MINUTES).

Chicken at Gratin

Ingredients

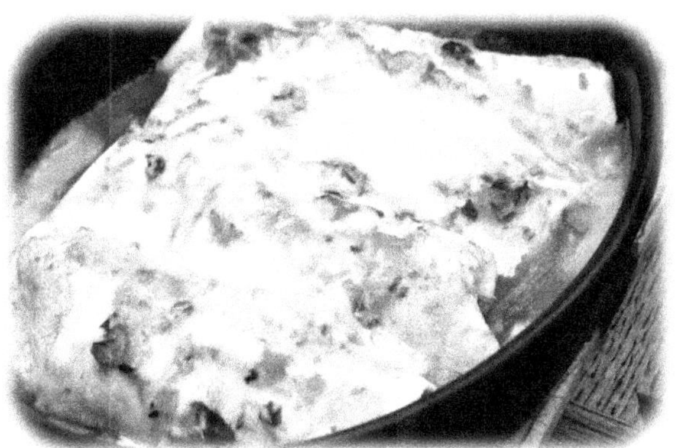

- 1 Chicken Breast
- 2 strips bacon, chopped
- Spicy Paprika
- 150g Cream Cheese
- 50g Cheddar Cheese
- 50g Mozzarella cheese
- ¼ Tabasco cup
- Salt and pepper

Preparation

Preheat the oven to 180°C. Season the chicken with salt, pepper and bake for 10 - 15 minutes. In a skillet over medium heat, add and sauté bacon until crisp. Add cream cheese, paprika, and Tabasco. Mix until homogenized, bathe the chicken and cover with the cheese. Bake for 8 - 10 minutes until au gratin. Serve hot with sliced avocado or salad.

Caprese Chicken

Ingredients

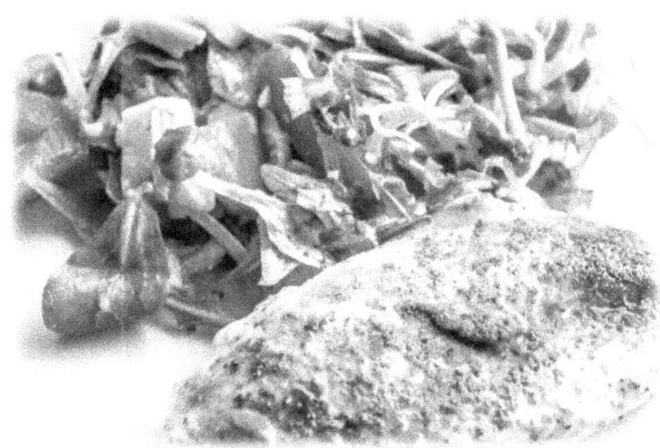

- 1 chicken thigh
- 1 tablespoon butter
- 3 quartered cherry tomatoes
- Grated mozzarella
- Fresh basil leaves
- Salt and Pepper

– Olive oil

Preparation

Season the chicken with salt and pepper and set aside. In a frying pan melt butter with oil, place the chicken and brown for 3 - 5 minutes per side. Remove from heat, cover and set aside. In a separate frying pan, place the oil and sauté the tomatoes together with the basil. Serve the chicken hot, cover with mozzarella and accompany with tomatoes.

Pepperoni Pizza in Skillet

Ingredients

– 2 cups mozzarella
– 1 cup almond flour
– ½ cup cream cheese
– 1 Egg
– Grated mozzarella
– Italian herbs and oregano
– Salt and pepper
– ½ cup tomato sauce
– 16 slices of pepperoni

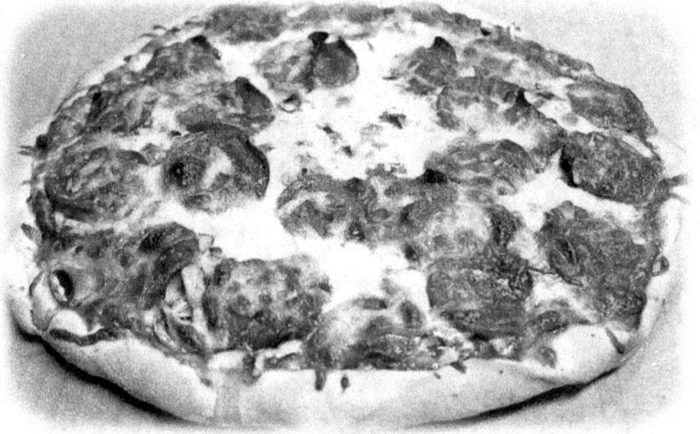

Preparation

In a skillet over low heat, place 2 cups cheese and stir until melted. Remove from heat, add cream cheese, egg and mix well. Add Italian herbs, almond flour, salt, and pepper, stirring until dough is formed. Stretch and place in a frying pan over medium heat. Cover and cook for 8 - 10 minutes. Turnover, add tomato sauce, grated mozzarella, pepperoni, oregano, cover and cook for 10 minutes. Serve hot

Meatballs in Tomato Sauce

Ingredients

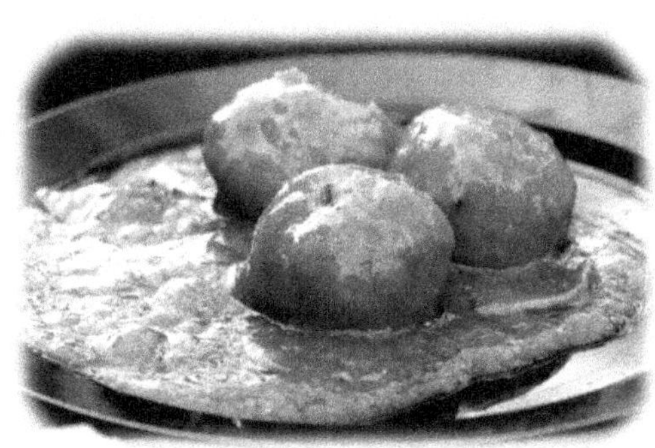

- ½Kg Ground beef
- 1 cup almond flour
- 2 chopped onions
- ½ Chopped paprika
- 100g Cilantro
- 4 cloves of garlic
- Salt and pepper
- Juice of 1 lemon
- Olive oil
- 800g Peeled tomatoes

Preparation

Preheat the oven to 180ºC. Process onion, paprika, cilantro, garlic, lemon juice, and olive oil until smooth. Add the meat and knead together with the almond flour, salt, and pepper to form dough. Form spheres, place them on a previously greased baking tray and bake for 5 - 7 minutes. Process and season the tomatoes and put them in a saucepan over medium heat until boiling. Add the meatballs to the sauce and cook for 5 - 7 minutes. Serve hot and accompany with quinoa or avocado salad.

Buffalo Cream Chicken

Ingredients

- 2 chicken breasts, chopped
- 1 finely chopped onion
- 3 Crushed garlic
- 100g Cilantro finely chopped
- 2 tablespoons butter
- ½ cup buffalo sauce
- 1 cups chicken broth
- 1 cup of milk cream
- Salt and Pepper

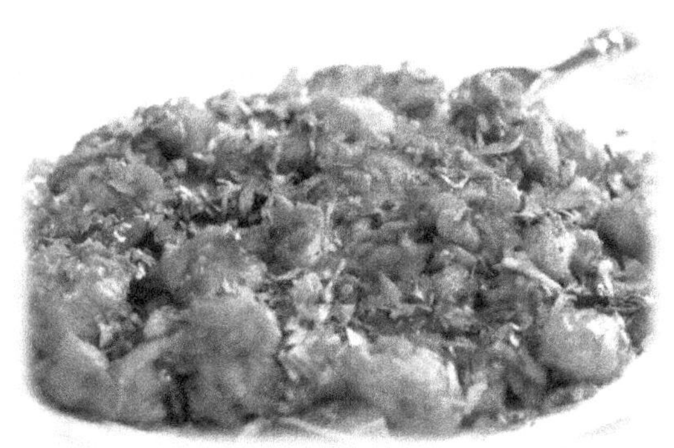

Preparation

In a skillet, heat over medium heat, add oil, chicken and sauté until golden brown. Remove from heat and set aside. In the same frying pan, melt the butter and oil over medium-high heat; add onion and garlic and sauté until golden brown. Add broth, salt, and pepper, buffalo sauce and bring to a boil. Add cream, chicken and cook until thickened. Remove from heat, sprinkle with cilantro and serve with red quinoa and salad.

Dill Salmon

Ingredients

- 1 salmon fillet
- Tarragon and Dill
- 1 teaspoon sesame oil
- Salt and pepper
- 1 tablespoon butter
- ¼ Cup of milk cream

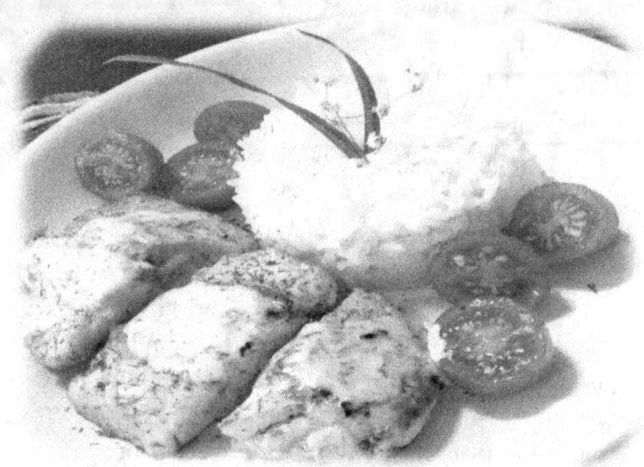

Preparation

In a frying pan over medium heat, add oil, salt, and pepper the salmon and place in the frying pan. Cook for 2 - 4 minutes per side, remove from heat, cover and set aside. In a frying pan melt the butter, add tarragon, dill and brown the butter. Add the cream and mix well until thickened. Serve the salmon covering with the sauce and accompany with a salad.

Tenderloin with Green Sauce

Ingredients

- 2 Loin medallions
- Soy sauce
- Salt and pepper
- Olive oil
- Juice of 1 lemon

- 4 Garlic
- 1 Chile, finely chopped
- 1 cup chopped cilantro
- Paprika
- ½ teaspoon cumin

Preparation

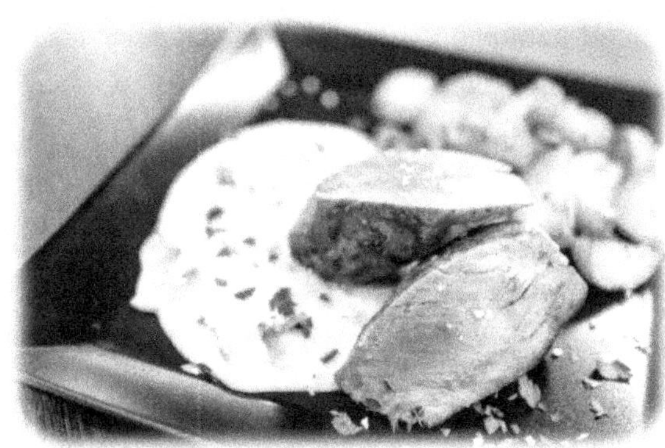

In a bowl place tenderloin, soy sauce, garlic, chili, mix well and leave to marinate for 1 hour in the refrigerator. In a skillet over medium heat, place oil and meat. Cook for 5 - 10 minutes per side, remove from heat, cover and set aside. Place cilantro, oil, lemon juice, paprika, cumin in the blender glass and process until a sauce is made. Serve the medallions hot, cover with cilantro sauce and accompany with quinoa or mashed cauliflower.

Mustard Filet

Ingredients

- 1 fish filet
- 1 tablespoon mustard
- 5 tablespoons vinegar
- Salt and pepper
- 1 tablespoon olive oil
- ½ finely chopped paprika
- ½ Onion, finely chopped

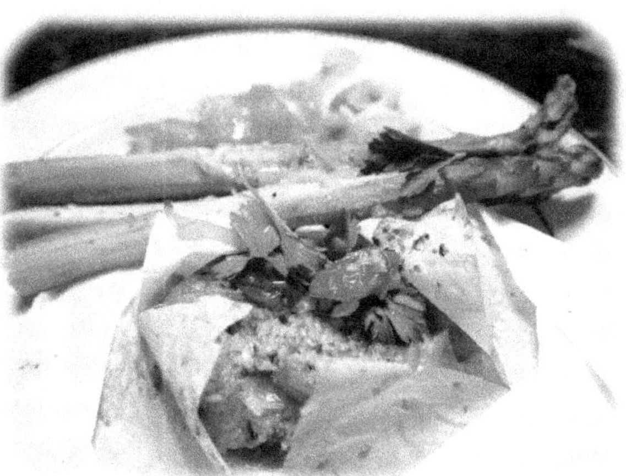

Preparation

Place the fish on aluminum foil, fold the edges of the paper upwards, spread the fish with mustard, jalapeño, vinaigrette and season with salt and pepper. Add onion, paprika, close like an envelope and 180°C for 12 - 16 minutes. Serve with salad or hard-boiled eggs.

Paprika Breast

Ingredients

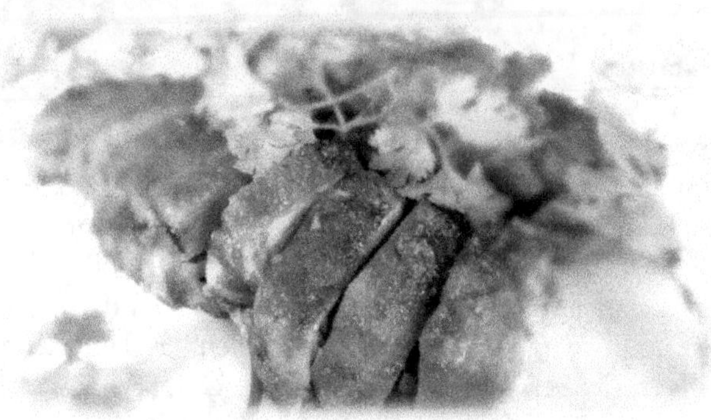

- 2 chicken breasts
- Olive Oil
- 2 tbsp Paprika
- Juice of 1 lemon
- 2 Crushed garlic
- Salt and Pepper

Preparation

Season the chicken with salt and pepper and set aside. In a bowl mix oil, paprika, lemon juice, garlic and bathe the chicken. In a hot skillet over medium heat, place oil, chicken and cook for 4 - 6 minutes per side. Serve hot with avocado salad and cauliflower puree.

Sautéed Ground Meat

Ingredients

- 400g Ground beef
- 1 finely chopped onion
- 1 Tomato, chopped
- 1 chopped paprika
- Paprika
- 2 Crushed garlic
- 1 tablespoon oregano
- 1 tablespoon chili powder

- Salt and pepper
- Cilantro finely chopped
- Coconut oil

Preparation

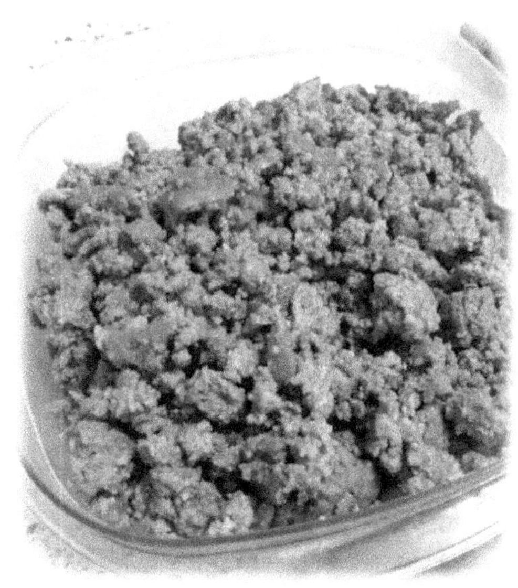

In the blender glass, adds tomato, paprika, garlic, and process. In a frying pan over medium heat place the choir oil, add onion and sauté until golden brown. Add the meat and sauté until it changes color. Add the liquefied, chili, oregano, paprika, salt, pepper, mix and cook. Remove from heat, add cilantro and serve hot, accompanied with quinoa or salad.

Meat with Spinach

Ingredients

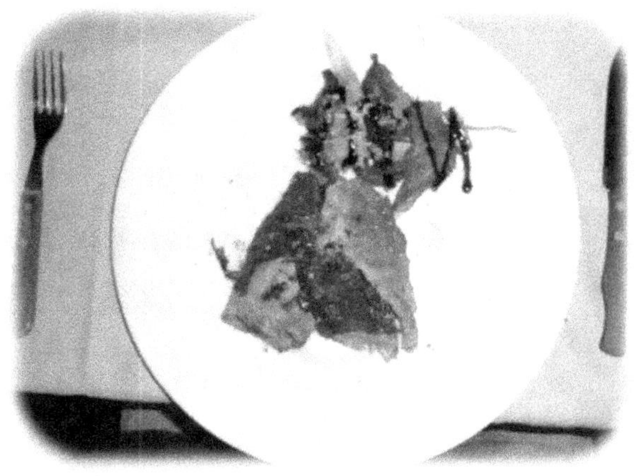

- 1 diced paprika
- Spinach leaves
- 300g Meat cubes
- 30g aioli sauce
- Olive oil
- Grated mozzarella
- Salt and pepper

Preparation

In a hot skillet over medium heat place oil, add meat and sauté until browned. Add paprika, aioli, salt, pepper, and mix for 4 - 8 minutes. Remove from heat, add spinach, mix and serve hot with quinoa or salad.

Cauliflower Spanish Tortilla

Ingredients

- 5 Eggs
- 2 finely chopped onions
- 1 Cauliflower, chopped
- Olive oil
- Salt and pepper

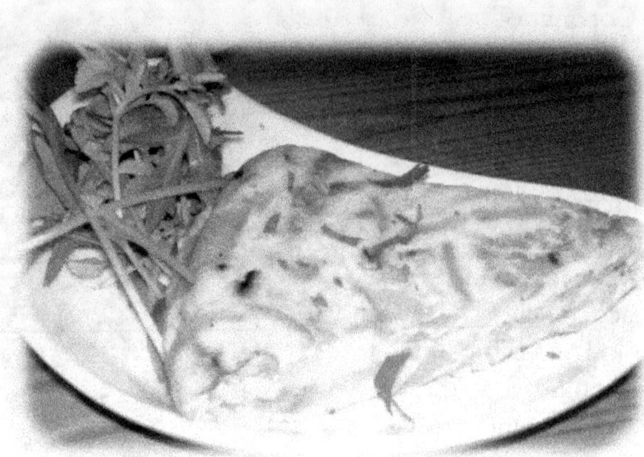

Preparation

In a pot of boiling water place the cauliflower and cook for 1 - 3 minutes. Remove from heat, drain and set aside. In a frying pan over medium heat, add oil, onion and sauté until golden brown. Add cauliflower and sauté until tender. Beat the eggs vigorously with spoonfuls of water, salt, and pepper. Add them to the frying pan, cover and cook until dry on one side. Turn over with the help of a plate and finish cooking. Serve hot with avocado cream and natural juice.

Cheese Omelet

Ingredients

- 2 Eggs
- 3 bacon strips
- 2 slices of cheese
- Salt and pepper
- Oregano
- Paprika

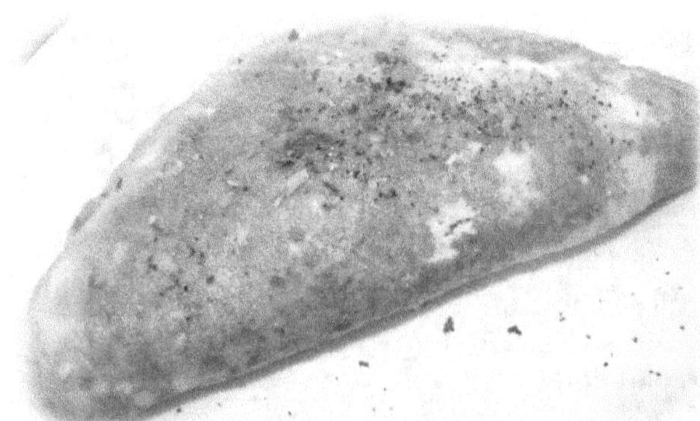

Preparation

Beat the eggs with salt, pepper, oregano, and paprika. In a frying pan over medium heat, place the bacon over medium heat until golden, remove from heat and set aside. In the same skillet over medium heat, pour a thin layer of egg and turn over. Add bacon, cheese, and close. Serve hot with avocado.

Pork Loin with Broken Eggs

Ingredients

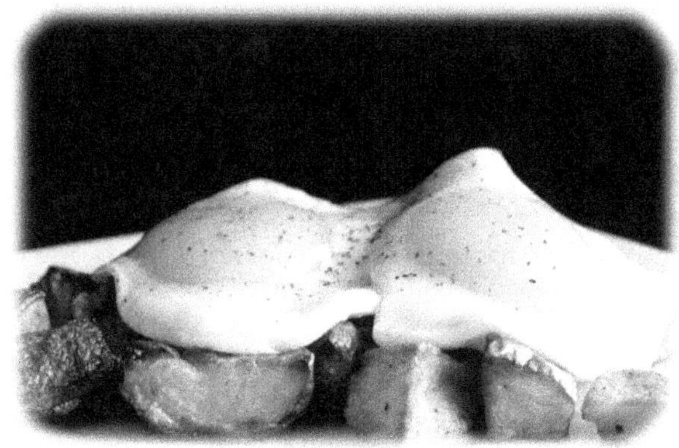

- 2 Eggs
- 300g Pork loin in cubes
- 1 tablespoon butter
- 3 Crushed garlic
- Cilantro finely chopped
- Salt and pepper
- Olive oil

Preparation

Season the meat with salt, pepper, garlic, and reserve. In a hot frying pan over medium heat, add oil, pork and sauté until golden brown. Reserve the meat and place the eggs in the same frying pan, season with salt and pepper, cover and cook until curdled. Serve the pork and put the eggs on top, breaking the yolk when serving.

Sauteed Cabbage

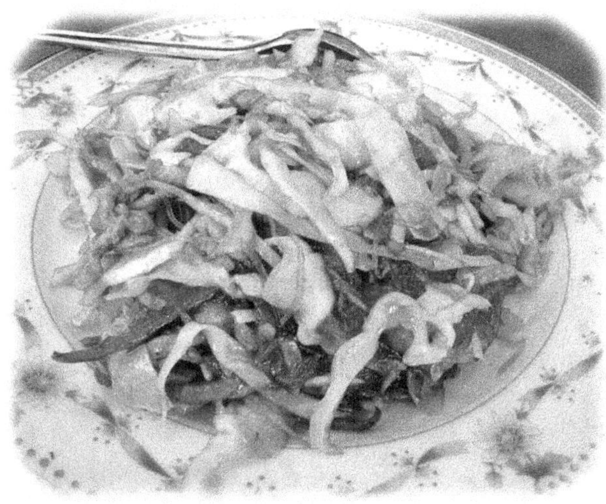

Ingredients

- 4 bacon strips
- 50g Chives, finely chopped
- 1 tablespoon butter
- 4 Eggs

- 100g grated mozzarella
- 1 grated cabbage
- Olive oil
- Salt and pepper

Preparation

In a skillet over medium heat, place bacon and cook until golden brown. Remove from heat and set aside. In the same frying pan over medium heat, melt the butter with olive oil, chives, cabbage, season with salt and pepper and sauté until golden brown. Beat the eggs with mozzarella, salt, pepper and pour into the frying pan. Mix and cook until dry. Chop the bacon and add it to the frying pan. Serve hot and accompany with quinoa.

Bacon and Chicken Salad

Ingredients

- 1 chicken breast, chopped
- 1 tablespoon butter
- 4 bacon strips
- 4 cherry tomatoes, halved
- 1 Washed lettuce
- Salt and pepper
- Olive oil
- 3 Eggs
- Juice of 1 lemon
- 3 Garlic

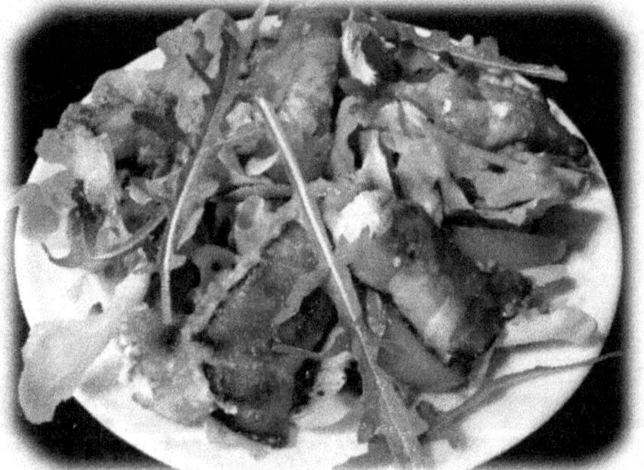

Preparation

Place eggs, lemon juice, garlic in the blender glass, process and slowly pour oil until thickened and reserved. Place bacon in a frying pan over medium heat and cook until golden brown. Remove from heat and set aside. In the same skillet over medium heat, melt butter with oil; add chicken and sauté until golden brown. Mix lettuce, tomato, chicken and bacon. Serve the salad with Quinoa, chicken, fish or meat.

Aioli Salmon

Ingredients

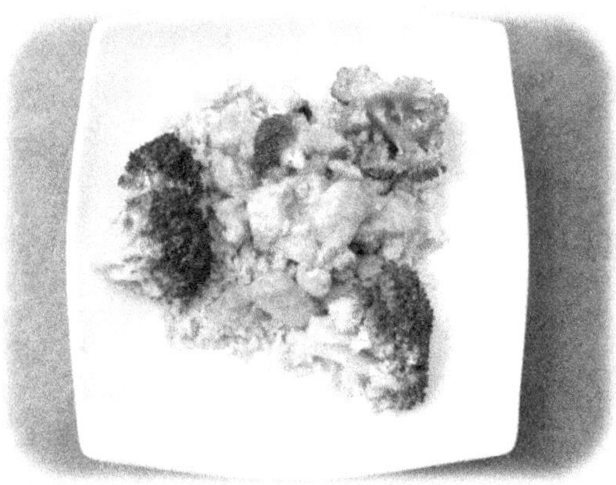

- 1 cup of Aioli
- Juice of 1 lemon
- 300g Salmon, chopped
- 2 tablespoons butter
- 1 Broccoli shelled
- Salt and pepper

Preparation

In a pot with boiling water place the broccoli and cook for 1 - 3 minutes. Mix aioli, lemon juice, salt, pepper and reserve in the refrigerator. In a hot frying pan over medium heat, melt the butter with oil, season the salmon, place it on the butter and sauté until golden brown. Add broccoli and sauté for 5 minutes. Serve hot with aioli and accompany with a salad.

Caprese Tortilla

Ingredients

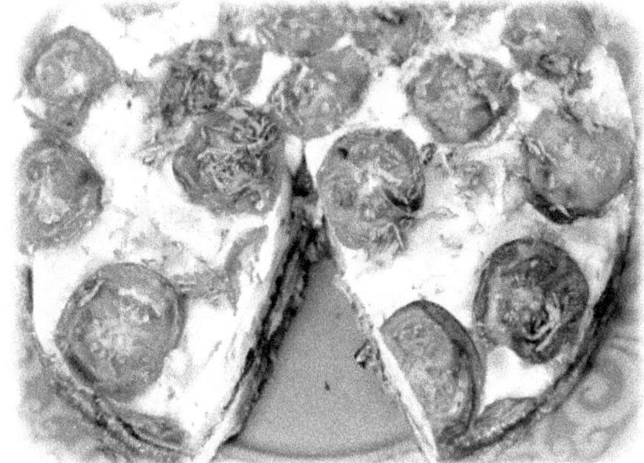

- Olive oil
- 4 Eggs
- 4 cherry tomatoes, halved
- Basil leaves
- Grated mozzarella
- Salt and pepper

Preparation

Beat the eggs with salt, pepper, 2 tablespoons of water, basil, cheese, tomato, and reserve. In a frying pan over medium heat place oil, pour all the mixture, cover and cook until dry on one side. Turn over with the help of a plate and finish cooking. Serve hot decorated with more basil.

Avocado with Aioli and Salmon

Ingredients

- 1 avocado
- 100g Smoked salmon
- 2 tablespoons aioli
- Salt and pepper
- Juice of 1 lemon

Preparation

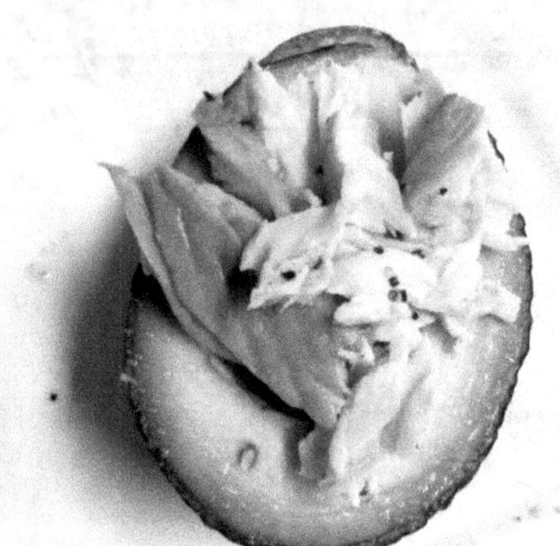

Cut the avocado in halves along the length and remove the stone, cleaning the halves. Varnish the halves with lemon, fill with aioli, salmon, salt, pepper and sprinkle more lemon. Serve fresh and accompany with quinoa.

Roasted Curry Chicken

Ingredients

- 2 shredded breasts
- 1 tablespoon curry powder
- 1 tablespoon garlic powder
- Coconut oil
- 1 Cauliflower shelled

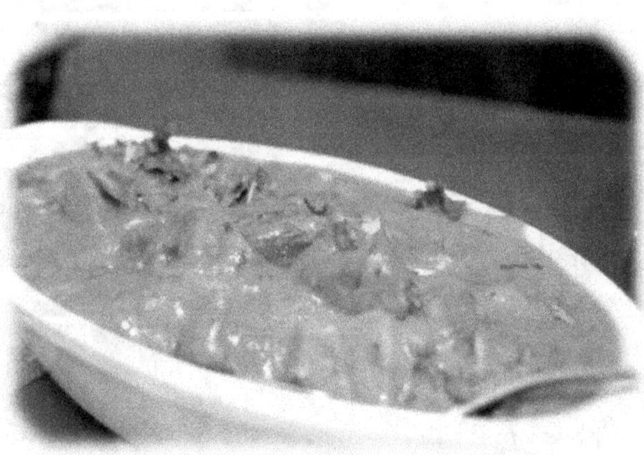

- 1 finely chopped paprika
- 200g Chicken broth
- Salt and pepper
- 100g finely chopped coriander

Preparation

In a pot of boiling water place the cauliflower, cook for 3 minutes, drain and set aside. In a skillet over medium heat, place coconut oil, curry, garlic and sauté until aromas are released. Add the chicken, season with salt and pepper and sauté until golden brown. Add cauliflower, paprika, broth and simmer for 10 - 15 minutes. Season, mix and serve to sprinkle with coriander.

Courgette Cake with Cheese

Ingredients

- 2 Courgettes in slices
- Olive oil
- 100g Cream cheese
- 100g grated mozzarella
- 1 finely chopped paprika
- 2 Eggs
- 1 finely chopped onion
- Finely chopped parsley
- Salt and pepper

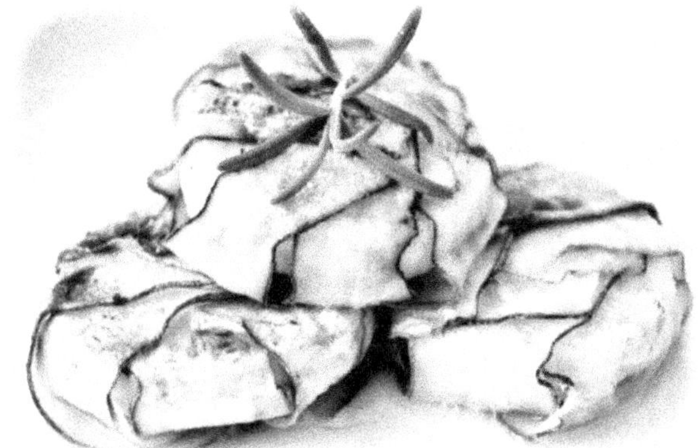

Preparation

Preheat the oven to 180°C. On a hot plate varnished with oil, place the zucchini, brown for a few minutes and set aside. In a frying pan over medium heat, put oil, onion, paprika and sauté until golden brown. Mix cheese, parsley, egg, sauté, salt, pepper, and reserve. On a previously prepared baking sheet, place a layer of zucchini, cover with the previous mixture, cover with the rest of zucchini and bake for 5 - 10 minutes. Serve hot with salad.

Spicy Chicken

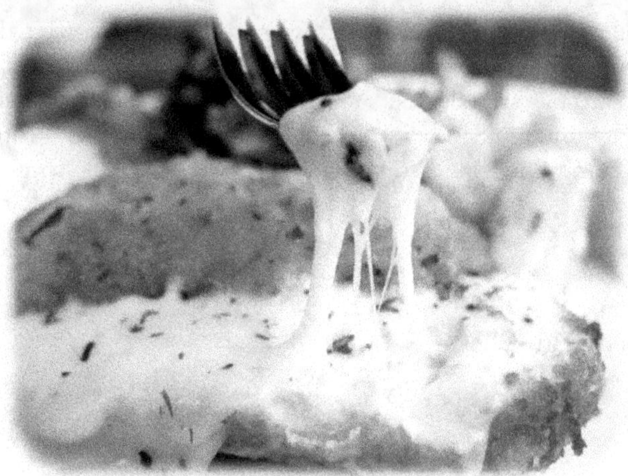

Ingredients

− 2 breasts
− Paprika
− Tabasco sauce
− Aioli sauce
− 150g Cheddar
− 50g Mozzarella
− 250g Cream Cheese
− Salt and pepper

Preparation

Preheat the oven to 180°C. Season the chicken, place in a bowl and mix with paprika, aioli, Tabasco, cream cheese and set aside for 5 - 10 minutes. Take to a previously prepared baking tray and bake for 20 - 30 minutes. Cover with cheese and bake for 5 - 10 minutes more. Serve hot and accompany with an avocado salad.

Broccoli Croquettes

Ingredients

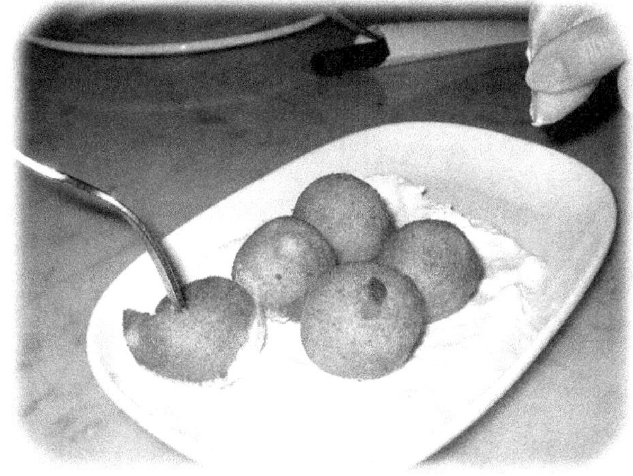

- 1 cup tapioca flour
- 1 broccoli
- 100g grated mozzarella
- 2 Eggs
- 1 tablespoon baking soda
- ½ cup cream cheese
- Salt and Pepper

Preparation

Preheat the oven to 180°C. In a pot of boiling water place the broccoli, cook for 1 - 3 minutes, drain and set aside. In a food processor add broccoli, flour, mozzarella, baking soda, egg, and process until firm dough is formed. Form spheres, place on a pre-prepared baking sheet and bake for 15 - 20 minutes. Serve hot with cream cheese.

Fish with Garlic Butter

Ingredients

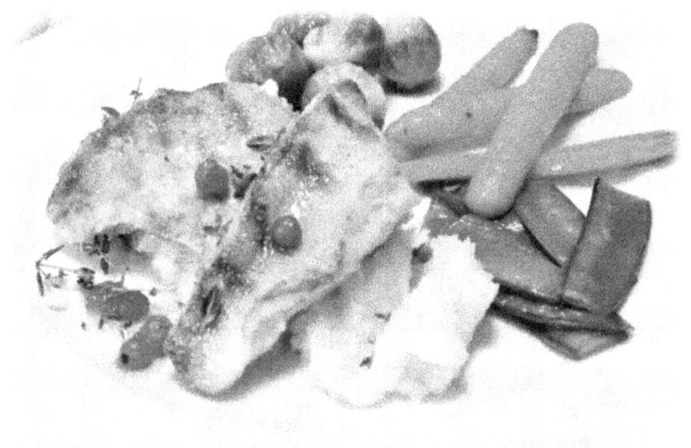

- 1 fish fillet
- 3 Crushed garlic
- 100g Parsley, finely chopped
- Olive oil
- 150g Butter
- Salt and pepper

Preparation

In a bowl add butter, parsley, garlic, salt, pepper, mix well and place on a piece of paper film. Roll up the film in the form of tobacco and keep in the refrigerator. Season the fish in a frying pan over medium heat, add oil and salmon. Cook for 2 - 5 minutes per side. Serve hot the fish accompanied by salad, Place on top slices of butter reserved in the refrigerator.

Medallions with Jalapeño Cream

Ingredients

- 3 Beef medallions
- Soy sauce
- Salt and pepper
- Olive oil
- 4 Garlic
- Paprika
- 1 cup cilantro
- 1 Jalapeño
- 200ml Milk cream

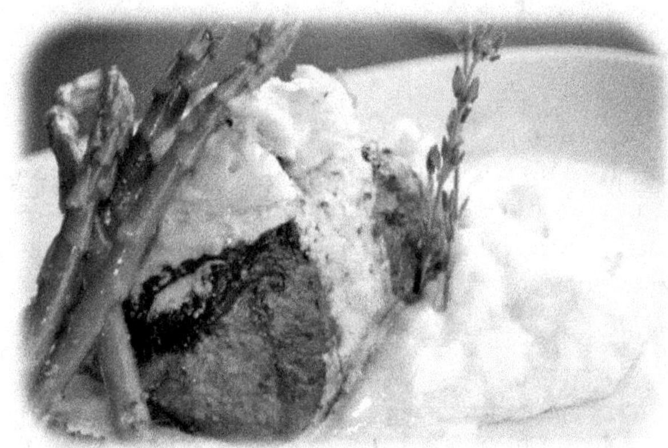

Preparation

In the blender glass, adds soy sauce, oil, paprika, cilantro, jalapeño, garlic, then process well until forming a sauce. In a bowl place the medallions, bathe with the sauce previously made and let macerate for 30 minutes. In a hot frying pan over medium heat, place the oil, the medallions and brown for 5 - 10 minutes per side. Remove from heat and set aside. Pour the macerated meat liquid into the frying pan and bring to the boil, season with salt and pepper and add cream, let it thicken and serve the meat hot, bathing with the sauce and accompanied with an avocado salad or cauliflower purée.

Stewed Pork

Ingredients

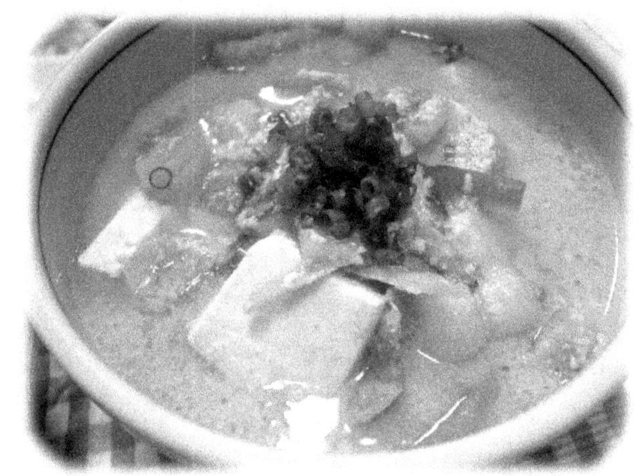

- 300g Pork, cut into pieces
- 3 Crushed garlic
- 3 finely chopped tomatoes
- 1 finely chopped onion
- 1 grated carrot
- 1 cup chicken broth
- Olive oil
- Salt and pepper

Preparation

Place oil, onion, garlic, carrot in a saucepan over medium heat and sauté until golden brown. Add pork and sauté until well browned. Add tomato, broth and bring to a boil. Season with salt and pepper and reduce to taste. Serve hot with quinoa.

Sautéed Quinoa

Ingredients

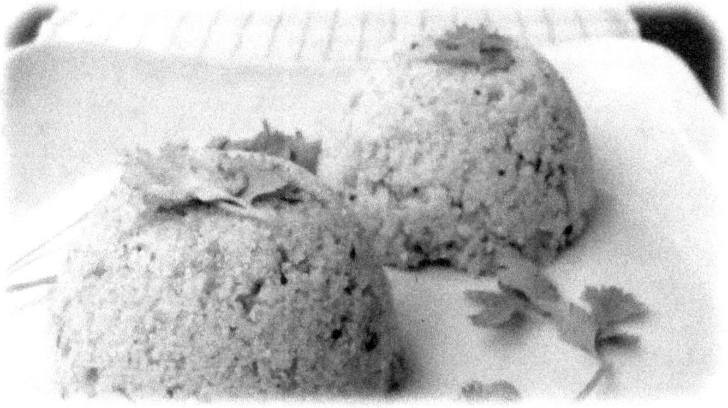

- 1 grated cabbage
- 1 finely chopped onion

- 2 finely chopped paprika
- 3 cups cooked quinoa
- 3 Crushed garlic
- Basil
- Olive oil
- 3 tablespoons soy sauce
- Salt and pepper

Preparation

In a wok over medium-high heat, place oil, onion, garlic and sauté until golden. Add cabbage and sauté for 5 minutes. Add quinoa, soy sauce, salt, pepper and sauté for 5 minutes. Finally, add basil and mix well for 5 minutes. Correct the salt and serve hot with salad.

Quinoa with Fish

Ingredients

- 1 fish filet, chopped
- 1 finely chopped onion
- 2 grated carrots
- 1 chopped paprika
- 3 Garlic
- 1 finely chopped leek
- Parsley
- 1 cup quinoa
- 1 Tomato
- 2 cups fish stock
- Olive oil
- Salt and pepper

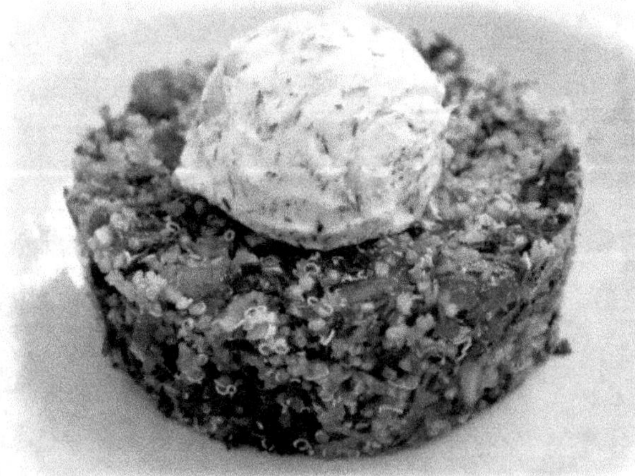

Preparation

In the blender glass, add garlic, paprika, carrot, leek, parsley, tomato, fish stock, salt, pepper, and process well. In a pot over medium heat, place oil, onion and sauté until golden. Add quinoa, fish, salt, pepper and sauté well. Add the liquefaction, mix, bring to a boil and cook over low heat for 20 - 25 minutes.

Cucumber Cream with Fine Herbs

Ingredients

- 2 chopped cucumbers
- 200g Diced cassava
- 1 chopped onion
- 100g grated mozzarella
- Olive oil
- Fine herbs
- Salt and pepper

Preparation

In a pot of boiling water with salt over high heat, place cucumber, yucca and onion for 10 - 15 minutes. Once the

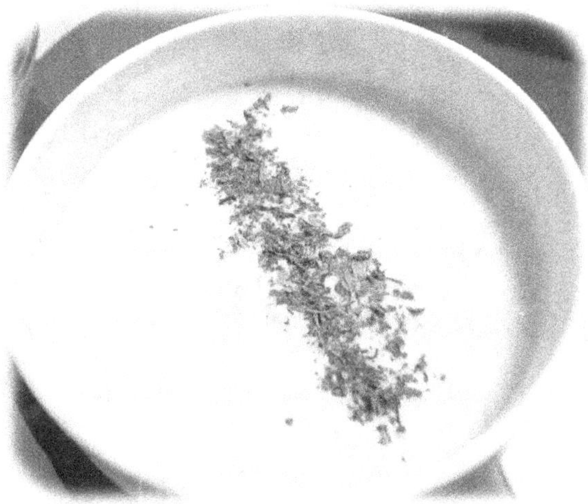

yucca is soft, process all the ingredients with the fine herbs in a blender, season if necessary and serve hot decorating to taste.

Duck Magret with Herbs

Ingredients

- 1 duck breast
- 1 tablespoon honey
- 3 tablespoons wine vinegar
- Butter
- Juice of 1 orange

– Italian Herbs
– Olive oil
– Salt and pepper

Preparation

In a bowl mix Italian herbs, orange juice, wine vinegar, honey, and oil.
Bathe the duck and reserve for 15

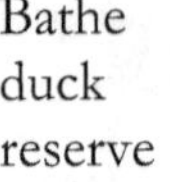

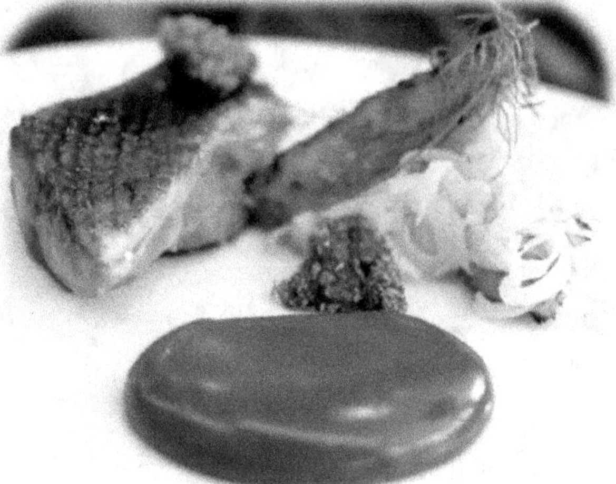

minutes. In a hot frying pan over medium heat melt butter with oil, place the magret and cook 10 - 12 minutes per side. Remove from heat and serve bathed with the sauce of preference, accompanied with quinoa or salad.

CHAPTER IX

TIPS

- Use olive, canola, coconut or avocado oils, preferably.
- Avoid the use of sweeteners.
- Be careful when consuming salt.
- Avoid fried foods.
- Use a carbohydrate calculator, if this is not possible, use a chart to help you, kitchen weight and measuring cup.
- Add a little butter to hot drinks like tea or coffee.
- Take sodium, potassium, and magnesium supplements.
- Drink plenty of fluids and stay hydrated throughout the day.
- Drink flavored water with lemon, the flower of Jamaica or another ingredient of natural origin.
- Complement main meals with green vegetables and legumes.
- Check the labels of medicines, many of them contain carbohydrates, which are counterproductive.
- Read labels on packaged foods to avoid those that contain carbohydrates.
- Avoid buying foods that are not allowed in the ketogenic diet.
- Empower the family by involving them in food selection and preparation.
- Prepare meals and keep frozen those that require longer cooking time, using food preservation techniques.
- Chew the food very well and rest after eating the food.
- If you consider yourself vegetarian or vegan, you can adopt the ketogenic diet, without problems.
- Avoid rewarding yourself with food.
- Read self-help books.

❖ **Plate Technique:** is a technique that produces a psychological effect and helps you control the amount of food when serving.

It consists of symbolically dividing a dish into 2 equal parts, then dividing one of the parts into 2 equal portions. Being distributed in 25%, 25% and 50% of the plate.

In the part of 50% serve green vegetables and vegetables with low carbohydrate content and plenty of fiber, in a section of 25% serve generous amount of foods rich in good fats and in the other section of 25%, serve protein.

CONCLUSIONS

The ketogenic diet comprises a set of elements that must be applied in a coordinated manner to obtain the expected results.

The correct selection and combination of foods, changing eating habits, knowing your own organism, physical activity and a firm decision to improve your life, are the main elements to ensure the success of this wonderful eating plan.

The body needs to get rid of the toxins that have accumulated over time; this is a process that is being carried out gradually, with a lot of discipline, organization, and responsibility.

Transforming your life is a process that starts from the inside out, starting with your mind, changing your lifestyle, to enjoy a full life, showing a clear mind in a healthy body.

You must have a clear goal of what you want to achieve, visualize an image of the person you want to become, following the advice contained in this EBook and fulfilling each of the objectives that lead you to success.

With the acquisition of this EBook, you have taken the most essential step in this process that will change your life, become your best friend and prepare for the enjoyment of a full life.